Nutrition and Pineal Development for Enhanced Performance and Sexual Wellness

A Three-Week Strategy to Boost Penile Wellness for Greater and More Intense Intimacy.

Phildeoner KT.

Contents Table

Chapter One

Overview

Distinguishing between generally held beliefs and realities backed by research becomes crucial in the huge subject of health and wellness, where information is abundant. Given the abundance of misconceptions and myths surrounding sexual health, this distinction is particularly significant. This non-fiction article explores the topic of diet-related misconceptions surrounding penile growth in an attempt to distinguish truth from false assertions.

People frequently encounter a multitude of information regarding sexual health, some of which is founded on scientific truths and some of which are simply myths. Sexual health is a very personal and delicate matter. Gaining a deeper comprehension of sexual health and its intricacies requires a commitment to evidence-based research. As we embark on our nonfiction journey, we hope to dispel any myths and clarify the truth about penile growth.

There is a common misconception that certain foods, like coconut water, cashew nuts, peanuts, pineapple, and apples, may have an impact on penis size. Nevertheless, this notion is not well-supported by scientific data. The following 1,500 words will address a wide range of dietary insights, investigate the hormonal and genetic factors that influence penile growth, promote body acceptance, and conclude with a hearty dinner that embodies the essence of a comprehensive approach to wellbeing. Our research is firmly based in non-fiction and makes use of reliable scientific data to guide readers through an exploration of the pros and cons related to sexual health. By navigating these realities and dispelling myths, we hope to empower people to approach talks about sexual health with discernment and to advance a more informed, enlightened perspective on the intricacies of the human body. Armed with the knowledge gained from empirical study, let's embark on an investigative journey to dispel the myths surrounding penile development.

1.1 Synopsis of Myths About Penile Growth

There are misconceptions in the public mind about the anatomy of men, namely the size and growth of the penis. Disinformation, cultural attitudes, and societal expectations frequently reinforce these errors. It is essential to critically examine these myths and lay the groundwork for our understanding using scientific evidence.

There are numerous accounts of diets having a miraculous effect on penile development. Nuts, peanuts, pineapple, cashew nuts, and coconut water have all been suggested as potential sources of a larger penis. But it's crucial to keep in mind that these claims are unsupported by credible scientific data.

Science says that during puberty, hormones and genetic factors mostly govern penile development. Food consumption does not directly correspond with an increase in penile size. As we navigate the web of myths surrounding penile growth, it is imperative that we dispel these illusions and emphasize the need of relying on knowledge that is founded in the truth.

Beyond the realm of science, cultural norms and expectations frequently serve as the basis for myths regarding penile development. Conversations about virility and masculinity have the potential to unintentionally reinforce these stereotypes and fabricate a story that places undue strain on individuals. The objective of this review is to examine these social and cultural aspects in order to draw attention to the need for a more informed and ·practical perspective on penile health.

By examining these beliefs related to penile growth, we can begin the process of dispelling them and promoting informed discussions about sexual health. Understanding that these claims lack empirical backing is essential to developing a more open, accepting, and knowledgeable viewpoint regarding the intricacies of male anatomy. We'll look more closely at the nutritional makeup of the highly recommended meals in the sections that follow, along with the effects of hormones and genetics on penile growth and the development of positive body image. This non-fiction study seeks to arm readers with the knowledge and abilities needed to distinguish fact from fiction and approach discussions on penile development with a well-founded understanding.

1.2 Evidence-based health information's significance

The overwhelming amount of recommendations, advice, and purported treatments in the rapidly expanding field of health and wellness could be crippling. In the midst of this abundance, it becomes clear that people need to rely on evidence-based health information as a guiding principle in order to avoid falling victim to misleading information and make educated decisions.

The core foundations of evidence-based health information include clinical investigations, data analysis, and rigorous scientific research. This process ensures that the provided data are substantiated by real facts and have been thorough scrutiny by the scientific community, rather than being merely anecdotal or based on subjective opinions.

The propagation of misconceptions and incorrect notions around health is a significant challenge in the digital age. These misconceptions can range from the seemingly harmless to the perhaps harmful, and they may have an impact on people's choices, behaviors, and even how they perceive their bodies. Evidence-based information is important because it may dispel these beliefs and provide consumers with a reliable compass to navigate the complex world of health advice. There is a larger need than anyplace else for evidence-based information when it comes to sexual health conversations. Because they are fueled by cultural beliefs and anecdotal evidence, myths regarding penile development can give rise to unjustified anxiety and irrational expectations. By emphasizing the value of evidence-based information, we hope to provide people the confidence and a strong foundation in knowledge they need to engage in these discussions.

A valuable defense against medical quackery is the evidence-based health information's ability to stand out in a world full of quick fixes and miracle therapies. A filter that helps consumers sort through the noise and prioritize material that has been scientifically confirmed is provided by an evidence-based approach, which may be applied to everything from dubious food fads to unproven supplements or unfounded claims about physical improvement.

What ultimately makes evidence-based health information so important is its capacity to empower individuals to make informed decisions about their health. Whether choosing lifestyle choices, embracing a balanced diet, or understanding the subtleties of penile growth, evidence-based knowledge provides a solid foundation for people to design their own route toward optimal health.

We highlight the importance of relying on information that is backed by data as we examine the topic of sexual health nonfiction. The sections that follow will delve deeper into this inquiry and include subjects including nutritional insights, genetic and hormonal implications on penile growth, and body acceptance. With each new revelation, the goal remains the same: giving readers the knowledge they need to navigate the difficult world of sexual health with assurance and confidence.

Chapter Two

Analyzing the Accused Foods

A number of foods have become well-known in the realm of diet recommendations and nutritional trends because of their purported ability to influence many aspects of health, including penile growth. There have been suggestions regarding almonds, cashew nuts, pineapple, apples, and coconut water as potential sources of larger penises. However, more investigation reveals that these claims have, at most, minimal scientific support.

Pineapple, with its high vitamin C content and the anti-inflammatory enzyme bromelain, is well known for its vibrant taste and potential health benefits. There is no evidence that consuming pineapples increases penile development, despite the fact that these nutrients are good for overall health.

Apples are regarded as a symbol of health due to its high fiber content, high vitamin C content, and antioxidants. There is no proof to support the theory that eating apples affects penile development, despite the fact that eating them as part of a balanced diet may benefit general health.

Cashew nuts are prized for their creamy texture and rich nutritional makeup that includes large amounts of protein, essential minerals, and monounsaturated fats. Although cashew nuts offer many health benefits, including heart health and satiety, the notion that they encourage penile development is untrue. Because of their high protein level, healthy fat content, and assortment of vitamins and minerals, nuts are a popular snack food. Notwithstanding their nutritional value, scientists cannot agree on their role in penile growth. All of these foods are healthy and can be part of a balanced diet, but it's critical to distinguish between the benefits they offer for general health and the assertions they make regarding their ability to influence penile growth. The lack of scientific evidence linking these meals to penile growth highlights the need of relying on evidence-based information when making dietary decisions.

2.1 A pineapple

A popular fruit choice, pineapple is renowned for both its distinct flavor and potential health benefits. It has a sweet flavor and a tropical appeal. Although this tropical delight is a rich source of essential nutrients, it's important to distinguish between its general nutritional value and any specific influence on penile growth—a claim that lacks scientific proof.

One of the nutritional benefits of pineapple is its high content of vitamin C. This essential antioxidant is necessary for immune system support, iron absorption facilitation, and skin health maintenance. There's no evidence that the vitamin C in pineapples encourages penile development, despite the fact that vitamin C is typically beneficial to health.

An further well-known component of pineapple is the anti-inflammatory enzyme bromelain. Research has been done on the potential benefits of bromelain for reducing inflammation and enhancing digestion. However, there is currently no hard scientific proof linking bromelain to penile development.

Pineapple is rich in vitamin B6, fiber, and manganese in addition to high concentrations of vitamin C and bromelain. These elements promote overall energy, a healthy digestive system, and strong bones. While incorporating pineapple into a balanced diet can boost nutritional variety, it has no direct effect on penile development.

Because pineapple has a high water content and promotes hydration, it's a tasty option. In addition, the fruit contains electrolytes, such potassium, which the body needs to keep its fluid balance in check. While maintaining proper hydration is crucial for overall health, there isn't much proof that it specifically affects penile development. In terms of nutritional insights, pineapple is definitely good for you. Its vibrant flavor and nutritious composition make it a valuable supplement to a well-rounded diet in general. However, given that there is currently inadequate scientific evidence to support assertions about its participation in penile growth, it is crucial to view these comments with caution.

In order to better understand the connection between diet and sexual health, we will investigate analogous claims regarding additional foods that are heavily marketed as we do more research-based examination. This will expose the complexities of penile growth.

2.2 Apple

Apples, with their natural sweetness and crisp texture, have become associated with health benefits, as evidenced by the proverb "an apple a day keeps the doctor away." Although apples are undoubtedly a good source of nutrients, it's important to look at the specific nutrients they contain and dispel any myths regarding their potential to aid in penile development.

Apples are renowned for having a high fiber content; one medium-sized apple can provide a significant portion of the required daily fiber intake. This dietary fiber supports digestive health, helps control weight by promoting a feeling of fullness, and generally improves heart health. However, there is no conclusive link found between the growth of penile tissue and its content.

Antioxidants, particularly flavonoids, which support the body's defense against oxidative stress, are abundant in apples. They also include vitamin C, which is widely recognized for boosting collagen synthesis and immune system strength. Antioxidants and vitamin C are typically necessary for optimal health, but there is no evidence that the ingredients in apples promote the formation of penile tissue.

Apples' high water content aids in the body's hydration and maintenance of a healthy fluid balance. They also include vital minerals, such as potassium, which is heart-healthy. However, there is no conclusive evidence linking mineral content, moisture content, and penile growth in apples.

In addition to specific nutrients, apples include a variety of vitamins and minerals, including manganese, vitamin B6, and vitamin K. In a varied and balanced diet, eating apples is a good method to support nutritional diversity and overall wellbeing. It's crucial to distinguish between apples' general health benefits and any specific effects on penile development, though.

Analyzing the nutrients in apples reveals that they are a nutrient-dense addition to a diet that is well-balanced. Fiber, antioxidants, and other vitamins and minerals are all beneficial to overall health. However, given that there is now little scientific evidence to support claims made regarding apples and penile development, it is crucial to approach them with caution.

2.3 Almonds

Cashew nuts, with their crispy texture and rich, buttery taste, are a popular snack and a nutritional powerhouse. Cashews are a nutrient-dense, high-fatty acid food that is beneficial to overall health, but there is no scientific proof that it influences penile growth.

Cashew nuts may include monounsaturated lipids, which are heart-healthy fats similar to those in olive oil. These fats help lower harmful cholesterol levels, which has been related to cardiovascular health. Monounsaturated lipids, which are heart-healthy but have no direct impact on penile development, are found in cashews.

Cashews are high in protein and include the amino acids needed for many bodily functions, such as muscle maintenance and repair. They also include essential vitamins like K, E, and B6, as well as minerals like copper, phosphorus, zinc, and magnesium. While these nutrients are necessary for overall health, there is no specific link between them and penile development.

Cashews include compounds such as zeaxanthin and selenium, which are examples of antioxidants that help protect cells from oxidative stress. Additionally, cashews have anti-inflammatory properties that enhance overall wellness. These traits, however, do not demonstrate a connection between cashew consumption and penile development.

Cashew dietary fiber helps maintain digestive health by promoting regular bowel movements and improving nutrition absorption. The high fiber content of cashews is beneficial to overall health but has no obvious effect on penile development.

Without a doubt, a healthy diet should include a significant amount of cashew nuts due to their high vitamin content. Together, protein, healthy fats, vitamins, and minerals support numerous aspects of overall health. Nevertheless, considering the lack of current scientific evidence to support claims regarding cashews and penile development, it's critical to approach these claims with realism.

Owing to their delectable taste and versatility, peanuts are currently a widely consumed snack and ingredient in numerous culinary traditions. Although rich in nutrients and beneficial for overall health, there is no scientific evidence linking peanuts to the development of penile structures.

Nuts high in protein, like peanuts, are a good source of essential amino acids needed for body building, repair, and general function. Although consuming peanuts might directly affect penile growth, this theory is unsupported by scientific data. Muscular strength is one of the many aspects of health that protein is crucial for.

Peanuts include a mix of heart-healthy monounsaturated and polyunsaturated fats. They also include a range of essential nutrients, including vitamin E, niacin, and folate, and minerals like potassium, phosphorus, and magnesium. Despite being found in peanuts, these minerals are not particularly beneficial to penile development, despite their general health benefits.

Nuts are a great source of dietary fiber that promote regular bowel movements and aid in the absorption of nutrients, both of which support digestive health. The high fiber content of peanuts is beneficial to overall health but has no particular effect on penile development.

One antioxidant that's associated with heart health is resveratrol, which can be found in peanuts. Their nutritional profile is further enhanced by phytosterols and other plant constituents. There is no evidence that peanuts cause penile enlargement, despite the health benefits of these components.

Nutritious and containing a range of proteins, healthy fats, vitamins, and minerals, peanuts can be a valuable addition to a well-balanced diet. However, given the lack of current scientific evidence to support claims regarding peanuts and penile development, it's critical to approach these claims with caution.

2.4 Water from Coconuts

Comprehending Its Ingredients: Renowned for its health benefits and delectable taste, coconut water is derived from green coconuts. It's a well-liked hydration beverage. There is no scientific evidence to establish a direct correlation between the growth of penile tissue and coconut water, despite the fact that it is a fantastic method to stay hydrated and contains key nutrients. The main draw of coconut water is its high water content, which makes it a great choice for hydration on the go. It also includes electrolytes that support the body's fluid balance, such as calcium, magnesium, sodium, and potassium. However, the electrolyte and hydration qualities of coconut water have no direct effect on penile development. Coconut water is a nutrient-dense drink that provides a range of vitamins and minerals. There are trace amounts of several nutrients, including vitamin C, potassium, magnesium, and manganese. While these components are generally beneficial to your health, there is no scientific evidence that consuming coconut water promotes the development of penile tissue. Cytokinins, one type of antioxidant found in coconut water, may shield cells from oxidative stress and enhance cellular health. There is little evidence that the antioxidants in coconut water cause penile development, despite their importance to overall health.

Coconut water is a fantastic substitute for other sugar-filled beverages for individuals who want a hydrating drink that is low in calories and natural sugars, unlike many commercial drinks. However, this characteristic has no direct bearing on the growth of the penis. Understanding the components of coconut water is crucial to appreciating its role as a hydrating beverage with added nutritional benefits. Although coconut water is a great source of essential nutrients and hydration, claims that it specifically affects penile development should be taken with a grain of salt as there is currently scant scientific evidence to back up these

claims.

Chapter Three

Puberty and Genetics: The True Factors

The two main components of the intricate web of human development that affect an individual's physical and sexual characteristics, including penile growth, are puberty and genetics. The genetic blueprint and the hormonal symphony of puberty orchestrate the body's transformation from infancy to sexual maturity, while environmental factors such as lifestyle and nutrition influence overall health.

Each individual's physical appearance is derived on their unique genetic composition, which they inherited from their parents. The appearance of multiple qualities is regulated by this intricate code, which affects not only physical characteristics but also the magnitude and period of developmental turning points, such as sexual maturation.

A period of profound hormonal changes begins with the onset of puberty, when the pituitary gland releases hormones that trigger the gonads to produce sex hormones. The primary hormone involved in men is testosterone. This hormonal symphony coordinates the development of secondary sexual features and, more importantly, the enlargement of the genitalia, particularly the penis.

During puberty, there is an increase in testosterone levels which leads to the enlargement of the testes and the growth of facial and body hair. Concomitantly, this hormone surge facilitates penile enlargement. Everybody experiences a unique growth spurt throughout puberty, which is mostly determined by their genetic composition.

It's critical to acknowledge that penile size naturally varies widely throughout individuals. Genetics and puberty-related hormonal changes both have an impact on this type. In order to dispel unrealistic expectations and encourage a good body image, it is imperative to recognize and embrace these common variations.

While genetics and puberty play a significant role in penile development, it's critical to dispel myths and misconceptions around what constitutes a "normal" or "ideal" size. The emphasis ought to be switched to understanding sexual development realistically and appreciating the diversity that exists in human nature.

The real causes of penile growth include hormone fluctuations during puberty and genetics. Managing the transition from infancy to sexual maturity requires accepting the varied genetic makeup and hormonal variations that make each individual unique. As our evidence-based inquiry develops, we will delve further into a number of sexual health-related topics and provide insight into the factors influencing wellbeing.

3.1 Penile Size Genetic Variables

The intricate characteristics of the male anatomy, such as penis size and dimensions, are primarily inherited traits passed down from one's parents. Although societal and cultural perspectives can lead to misconceptions about what is "normal," a thorough understanding of human variation must consider the influence of genetics on penile size.

Genetic information inherited from both parents mostly determines physical traits. This blueprint contains a number of details, including height, facial traits, and—above all—genital measurements. The genetic material inherited from both parents shapes the spectrum of possible penile sizes for an individual.

Penile size is a polygenic characteristic, which means that a variety of genes can impact it. This complexity arises from the interaction of multiple genetic factors, each of which has a distinct effect on the growth and development of the penis. It becomes challenging to predict the precise outcome due to the intricate interaction of hereditary elements.

Genetic variability causes individuals to differ greatly in the range of penile diameters considered usual. It's important to realize that this diversity is entirely normal and the result of intricate interactions between genetic factors. People often miss the vast array of inherited typical differences when they measure themselves against unreachable norms or cultural objectives.

Penile growth is influenced by hormones and environmental factors, but DNA still lays the foundation for it. Penis development is largely influenced by hormonal changes during puberty and genetic predispositions. The expression of these inherited traits may vary based on environmental factors such as overall health and nutrition.

Debunking myths around penile size requires acknowledging and accepting the part heredity plays in defining individual differences. It's important to acknowledge that there isn't a one, widely agreed-upon notion of what constitutes a "ideal" size. Accepting genetic heterogeneity as a normal aspect of human nature is crucial for dispelling unrealistic expectations and fostering a positive body image.

The majority of penile size is determined by genetics. Together with hormonal and environmental variables, these polygenic traits explain why people come in such a wide range of sizes. We must recognize and celebrate this genetic variance in order to promote a healthy understanding of sexual anatomy and to value each person's uniqueness.

3.2 Hormonal Shifts During Adolescence

Puberty is a period of substantial change in human development, characterized by a series of hormonal changes that regulate the body's progression from childhood to sexual maturity. Variations in the endocrine system impact many aspects of mental and physical health as well as secondary sexual attributes and fertility. Robust feedback mechanisms regulate these oscillations.

Puberty is brought on by the complex interplay between brain and reproductive organ regulatory regions, or the hypothalamus-pituitary-gonadal (HPG) axis. The pituitary gland releases gonadotropin-releasing hormone (GnRH) in reaction to the brain releasing luteinizing hormone (LH) and folicle-stimulating hormone (FSH).

LH and FSH then activate the gonads, which are the testes in men and the ovaries in women, to produce sex hormones. Males mostly produce testosterone, whereas females produce oestrogen and progesterone. Physical and emotional changes brought on by elevated sex hormone levels are hallmarks of puberty.

An increase in testosterone production during male puberty results in the formation of an Adam's apple, deepening of the voice, and growth of facial and body hair. It also encourages the growth of the penis and testicles. In females, estrogen promotes the development of breast tissue, the onset of menstruation, and the expansion of the hips.

Hormonal changes during puberty are the main cause of growth spurts. Both sexes grow taller rapidly, with different puberty periods denoting the fastest growth. Sex hormones also influence bone growth, which ensures the attainment of skeletal maturity.

Hormonal changes associated with puberty are mediated by the adrenal glands. They produce adrenal androgens, which facilitate the growth of pubic and axillary hair. However, excessive testosterone can lead to acne, a serious concern during adolescence.

Hormonal fluctuations throughout puberty impact not only physical changes but also emotional and behavioral aspects. Adolescents may experience mood swings, increased emotional sensitivity, and changed social dynamics. Hormones and the developing brain interact to produce these changes in psychology.

It's critical to realize that every person goes through puberty at a different period and to a different degree. Genetic, environmental, and dietary factors all have an impact on these variations. Puberty may arrive for some persons earlier or later than it does for their peers.

Understanding the nuances of hormonal changes during puberty is crucial to being able to empathize with and support teens as they navigate this transformative stage of their lives. A thoughtful and positive approach to adolescent development and puberty is made possible by recognizing the variety of experiences and promoting candid discussion about these transitions.

3.3 Foods and Penile Growth Do Not Correspond

The assumption that specific diets affect penile growth is one of the many myths and misconceptions regarding sexual health. However, it's critical to disprove the notion that food choices directly affect the size of the penis. Since there is no consistent scientific evidence linking specific diets to penile growth, it is imperative to separate fact from fiction.

Penile size is mostly determined by hormones, particularly those associated with puberty, and genetics. The foundation for physical development is set by genetic information inherited from parents, and the growth of the genitalia, especially the penis, is mostly determined by hormonal changes throughout puberty that are mediated by the hypothalamus-pituitary-gonadal axis.

Despite what many people think, there are no miracle foods or dietary supplements that may change a person's genetic makeup or the hormones that control penile growth. Genetics plays a major role in determining the size and dimensions of the penis; statements to the contrary are not supported by scientific evidence.

Although a person's overall health and weight can affect their overall well-being, including their hormonal balance and cardiovascular health, there is no proof that body fat or any particular diet is directly linked to the development of penile tissue. Claims that specific meals might increase virility or grow the penile organ are frequently based more on false information than on scientific facts.

Believing that certain meals are effective in promoting penile growth might lead to inflated expectations and have a detrimental effect on one's self-esteem and body image. In order to recognize that variation in penile size is perfectly natural, it is imperative that correct information be disseminated and a healthy understanding of sexual anatomy be fostered.

Even if certain meals might not have an impact on penile growth, eating a healthy, well-balanced diet is important for general wellbeing. Foods high in nutrients support hormonal balance, cardiovascular health, and general wellbeing. It makes more sense to focus on eating a diet that promotes overall health rather than looking for items that are said to promote penile growth.

It is crucial to foster scientific literacy and critical thinking in order to navigate the deluge of false information surrounding sexual health. People ought to have access to reliable information so they may make decisions based on the evidence rather than giving in to peer pressure or unsubstantiated assertions.

The lack of a relationship between particular foods and penile growth emphasizes how crucial it is to trust scientific research and comprehend the complex processes that influence sexual development. A more realistic and constructive attitude to sexual health and well-being is ensured by separating myths from reality.

Chapter Four

Positive Body Image and Self-Acceptance

The concepts of body positivity and self-acceptance have grown to be powerful counterweights in a world where unachievable beauty standards and societal norms are ubiquitous. People may now celebrate and accept their bodies in spite of social norms because to these movements, which is changing how people view various bodies and making it more inclusive and caring. This is a deeper dive into the core concepts of body positivity and self-acceptance.

All bodies are valued and deserving of acceptance, regardless of size, shape, or appearance, according to the fundamental principles of body positivity. It challenges the idea of the ideal body type and emphasizes the uniqueness and beauty found in every individual. By encouraging people to value and celebrate the diversity of bodies, the movement fosters inclusivity and tolerance in society.

Media and advertisements frequently propagate cultural ideals of beauty, which can breed irrational expectations and body dissatisfaction. Body positivity, which holds that attractiveness is not restricted to a given size, shape, or skin tone, challenges these standards. It encourages a broader and more authentic representation of bodies in the media in order to promote acceptable expectations.

One needs to have a loving and understanding relationship with their body in order to be self-acceptant. It assists people in shifting their focus from supposed flaws to their body's strengths, resilience, and overall well-being. Self-love becomes a vital skill to deal with societal demands and retain a positive viewpoint.

Physique shaming is the act of criticizing someone's appearance or physical attributes. This is strongly opposed by body positivity. Whether it happens in person or online, body shaming promotes judgmental attitudes and unfavorable stereotypes. The movement aims to create a friendly environment where people can feel safe and accepted without fear of judgment.

In order to be inclusive, body positivity recognizes that a range of overlapping qualities, including ability, gender, ethnicity, and more, have an impact on perceptions of body image. The aforementioned declaration emphasizes the importance of acknowledging and addressing the unique challenges faced by individuals with diverse identities, ensuring that the movement is welcoming and supportive of everyone.

Media literacy is crucial for the body positive journey. Being aware of how the media affects people's perceptions of beauty empowers individuals to challenge overly dramatic portrayals and make informed choices. Encouraging people to scrutinise and evaluate media messages fosters a sense of agency in crafting their personal body narrative.

Building a support system is not only a personal journey but also a crucial component of body acceptance. Creating spaces where people can talk about their successes, setbacks, and experiences fosters a sense of belonging. Online forums and grassroots initiatives have played a significant role in fostering connections and creating communities centered around body positivity.

Body positivity and self-acceptance are at the core of a paradigm shift in how society views and values bodies. These movements contribute to the creation of a more compassionate and accepting society where people of all shapes and sizes can thrive by encouraging self-love, accepting diversity, and challenging harmful norms.

4.1 Fostering a Positive Self-Image

Promoting a positive body image requires nurturing a realistic and healthy perspective of one's own body, free from harmful self-criticism or erroneous social expectations. It's a process of coming to terms with who you are, appreciating your body for what it is, and embracing your uniqueness. The following are crucial pointers and strategies for promoting positive body image:

Encouragement of Self-Reflection:

- Inquire about people's thoughts regarding their physical appearance.

- Encourage self-awareness about how society affects how one feels about their body.

Impending Ideals of Impractical Beauty:

- Discuss and refute cultural beauty standards, which perpetuate limited ideas about what makes one attractive.

- Stress the diversity of beauty present in all racial and ethnic groups, age groupings, physical forms, and ability levels.

Promotion of Media Literacy:

- Learn the abilities required to evaluate images and messages seen in the media critically.

- Insist on the significance of diverse and realistic representations in the media.

Honoring Diversity of Body:

- Emphasize different body representations in advertising, fashion, and the media.

- Honor bodies in all shapes, sizes, and capacities.

Encouraging Well-Being Physically:

- Shift the focus from appearances to overall health.

- Promote a healthy lifestyle that includes regular exercise, a balanced diet, and adequate sleep.

How to Promote Compassion for Oneself:

- Encourage compassion and love for oneself.

- Discuss the significance of treating oneself with the same respect as one would a friend.

Constructing Communities of Support:

- Create communities that value support and diversity highly.

- Promote safe spaces for frank discussions on matters pertaining to body image.

Encouraging Self-Talk with Confidence:

- Encourage positive self-talk and affirmations for yourself.

- Help people reframe negative self-perceptions about their bodies into more constructive language.

Photoshop education and filters:

- Call attention to how ubiquitous picture editing and filters are on social media.

- Encourage sincerity and challenge the notion of "perfect" photographs.

Responding to Body Shaming:

- Create an environment that fiercely opposes physical humiliation.

- Encourage people to express their disapproval of behaviors and statements that disparage the body.

Promoting Mental Well-Being:

- Recognize the connection between mental health and body image.

- Encourage people to have access to mental health resources if they are experiencing physical issues.

Teaching Resilience and Coping:

- Provide tools to enable people to withstand social pressure and develop resilience.

- Provide healthy coping strategies to address stress and stressors associated with negative body image.

Including Adequate Behavior Models:

- Bring attention to positive role models that encourage and value a variety of body shapes.

- Honor those who prioritize their efforts and successes over appearances.

To encourage a positive body image, a multifaceted approach involving social, interpersonal, and individual efforts is required. By promoting self-acceptance, challenging harmful norms, and creating supportive environments, we contribute to the development of a culture where everyone may appreciate and love their physical appearance.

4.2 Fostering Acceptance of Oneself

Encouraging self-acceptance involves appreciating one's uniqueness and forging a positive relationship with oneself. It is a life-changing process. It's about not letting inflated social expectations get in the way of accepting one's own characteristics, idiosyncrasies, and defects.

The fundamental principles and strategies for promoting self-acceptance are as follows:

Accepting Personal Distinctiveness:

- Honor and acknowledge each person's uniqueness.
- Stress the value of diversity in terms of appearance and personality.

Constructing Self-Awareness:

- Urge people to reflect on their objectives, principles, and areas of strength.

- Promote self-awareness to understand boundaries, inclinations, and desires.

Rejecting Social Expectations:

- Condemn the unrealistic standards society has for attractiveness and prosperity.

- Promote the idea that a person's worth isn't solely determined by other people's opinions.

Building a Positive Self-Image:

- Promote activities that increase one's sense of value and self-esteem.

- Encourage others to focus on their abilities, accomplishments, and admirable qualities.

Develop Your Self-Compassion:

- Stress the importance of treating oneself with kindness and compassion.

- Emphasize the value of self-compassion as a practical tactic for overcoming setbacks and disappointments.

Splitting the Focus from Perfection:

- Emphasize that aiming for perfection is an unrealistic goal that cannot be accomplished.

- Encourage a mindset that places an emphasis on growth, advancement, and experience-based learning.

Boosting Confidence in Oneself:

- Help people recognize and stop talking to themselves negatively.

- Teach students how to replace negative words with phrases that are uplifting and reassuring.

Encouraging Self-Care:

- Promote self-care practices that prioritize one's mental, emotional, and physical well.

- Emphasize the need of setting boundaries and scheduling personal time.

Developing a Growth Mentality:

- Adopt a mindset that embraces challenges and sees failures as opportunities for improvement.

- Encourage a mindset that views personal development as an ongoing process.

Recalling Achievements and Significant Events:

- Honor each small but significant life achievement you have made.

- Create a culture where progress and hard work come before perfection.

Creating a Happy Environment:

- Encourage people to form trustworthy relationships.

- Promote environments that are upbeat, compassionate, and welcoming.

Setting Reasonable Goals:

- Help individuals set reasonable and meaningful goals.

- Give labor and growth greater weight than external measures of achievement.

Seeking Professional Help:

- Make it common practice to seek professional help when needed.

- Provide details about mental health choices and counseling services.

Typical Leadership Behavior:

- Set a positive example for self-acceptance and positive self-talk.

- Encourage others by sharing your own experiences of growth and self-awareness.

Building a loving and caring relationship with oneself is a necessary and effective step in promoting self-acceptance. By promoting these principles, we assist individuals in developing into strong, sincere individuals who embrace their uniqueness and take on life head-on.

4.3 Accepting the Natural Variety of Body Shapes

Accepting and celebrating the inherent diversity in body shapes is a necessary part of embracing the vast range of physical forms that occur among humans. It's a break from rigid beauty standards that uphold a narrow ideal and an acknowledgment of the range of sizes, forms, and proportions of bodies. The following are crucial pointers and strategies to promote acceptance of the wide range of natural body types:

Respecting Individuality:

- Reaffirm that every body is unique and lovely in its own way.

- Motivate individuals to appreciate their distinct features and characteristics.

Rejecting Idealized Standards:

- Challenge the notion of the "ideal" body shape that is promoted by society conventions and the media.

- Call attention to the harm caused by pushing unattainable, artificial beauty standards.

Displaying a Range of Representations:

- Promote diverse body images in the media, fashion, and advertising.

- Encourage the participation of individuals with a variety of body types to more accurately reflect the diversity found in the real world.

Creating Inclusive Spaces:

- Promote environments that respect and embrace a variety of body shapes.

- Take action against workplace and public discriminatory behaviors that involve body shaming.

Encouragement of Positive Phraseology:

- Promote the use of affirming and inclusive language when discussing bodies.

- It should be forbidden to use derogatory language or terms that support unfavorable body stereotypes.

Promoting Health at Every Size:

- Emphasize the importance of prioritizing your general health versus striving to fit into a specific body type.

- Bust the misconception that a person's looks are the only thing that determines their health.

Motivating Exercise for Positive Body Image:

- Participate in and encourage body positivity initiatives that celebrate and advocate for all body shapes.

- Distribute information and resources that bolster body-positive narratives.

Teaching Genetics and Body Shapes:

- Inform people on how heredity affects the forms of their bodies.

- Emphasize how a person's genetics, metabolism, and lifestyle all contribute to their individual body composition.

Encouraging Static Equilibrium:

- Encourage body neutrality by prioritizing practical skills over outward looks.

- Promote a positive, body-positive relationship that goes beyond appearances.

Promoting Fashion's Inclusivity:

- Support businesses and designers who prioritize inclusion in their sizing and marketing.

- Encourage a diverse range of body shapes to be featured in fashion advertisements.

Taking On Stereotypes in Fitness and Sports:

- Debunk rumors about the physical attributes of athletes and fitness.

- Encourage a more hospitable mindset that values and respects the diversity of bodies that engage in physical exercise.

Having Positive Discussions:

- Initiate and participate in conversations that promote diversity and positive body image.

- Tell personal stories and anecdotes that highlight the qualities that make different body forms attractive.

Promoting Body-Sustaining Initiatives:

- Support initiatives and organizations that work to promote inclusivity and body positivity.

- Take part in campaigns to dispel harmful beauty standards in order to raise awareness.

Accepting the natural diversity of body forms is one of the best strategies to create a more accepting and inclusive society. By opposing unrealistic expectations, promoting positive language, and celebrating individuality, we contribute to the development of a culture that cherishes and acknowledges the uniqueness of every body.

Chapter Five

Recipe for Honey-Glazed Pineapple and Nut Medley

Three-Weeks Nutrient-Rich Diet: Honey Glazed Pineapple and Nut Medley Smoothie Bowl

Parts:

One cup of unsweetened coconut flakes, half a cup of honey, four cups of fresh pineapple chunks, two cups of cashew nuts, two cups of peanuts, four tablespoons of coconut oil, and two pinches of crushed cinnamon

Optional ice cubes: 1 teaspoon sea salt

Directions:

Day 1–7 of Week 1: Morning Boost Smoothie Bowl

1. Combine the Foundation:

Put 2 cups fresh pineapple pieces, 1/2 cup coconut flakes, 1 cup cashew nuts, and 1 cup peanuts in a blender.

Blend until mixture is lump-free.

2. Attain Sheen and Display:

To prepare the honey-cinnamon glaze, melt 2 tablespoons coconut oil and whisk in 1/4 cup honey, 1 teaspoon ground cinnamon, and 1/2 teaspoon sea salt. Stir well.

Pour the glaze into the blender along with the pineapple and nut mixture. Stir for a short while.

Transfer into a dish, sprinkle with parsley if desired, and have your nutrient-rich morning boost!

First Week:

Bowl of Evening Indulgence Smoothie

1. Mix the Basis:

To guarantee a satisfying and delicious end to your day, make the smoothie bowl recipe from the morning again in the evening.

Weeks 2:

Continue as usual but add variation

1. Combine the Base:

Make smoothie bowls in the morning and evening using the same recipe, just with a few little adjustments, like adding ice cubes for a refreshing touch.

Week Three:

Final Week of Refueling, Days 15–21

1. Mix the Base:

Follow the plan and prepare your nutrient-dense ingredients

for the smoothie bowls in the morning and at night.

2. Think Back on Your Experience:

Ponder how this nutrient-dense program has improved your

overall well-being.

Additional Guidance

If you feel that eating the smoothie bowl twice a day is too

much, consider incorporating it into your routine once a day

or more frequently as it suits you.

Verify that the ingredients fit your dietary needs, and see a healthcare professional if you have any questions.

This nutrient-dense, three-week program is meant to be a nice and healthy addition to your daily routine. It includes a delicious and nutritious Honey-Glazed Pineapple and Nut Medley Smoothie Bowl. Let's toast to embarking on a healthy lifestyle!

5.1 Components

Recipe for a Nutrient-Rich Smoothie Bowl:

1. Four cups of newly chopped pineapple:

abundant in vitamins and enzymes that promote overall health.

2. A pair of cups cashew nuts:

plenty of healthy fats, protein, and essential minerals.

3. Two mugs of peanuts:

Packed with protein, fiber, and an assortment of vitamins and minerals.

4. One cup of coconut flakes without sugar added:

They offer a bit of tropical flavor along with healthy fats.

5. Half a cup of honey:

naturally provides sweetness and can have health benefits.

6. Four tsp raw coconut oil:

provides a good source of fats and a silky texture.

7. Two tablespoons of cinnamon powder:

This adds a toasty, aromatic flavor that enhances the flavor.

8. A tsp of sea salt:

provides a blend of taste and essential minerals.

For an Energizing Lifestyle

9. Ice cubes not required but optional:

Boost the texture and refreshing value of the smoothie.

Note: Because of their delicious flavor and potential health benefits, these items were chosen for the smoothie bowl. * Even though they might be a part of a balanced diet, each person has unique nutritional needs, so if you have any specific health concerns or dietary restrictions, it's better to consult a healthcare professional.

5.2 Actions

How to Make a Nutrient-Rich Pineapple and Nut Smoothie Bowl with Honey Glaze:

Day 1–7 (First Week): Boost Smoothie Bowl in the Morning

1. Blend in the Morning:

In a powerful blender, combine 2 cups fresh pineapple chunks, 1 cup cashew nuts, 1 cup peanuts, and 1/2 cup coconut flakes.

Blend until a smooth consistency is reached.

2. Preparing the Glaze:

Melt two tablespoons of coconut oil in a small skillet over low heat.

To the heated coconut oil, add 1/4 cup honey, 1 teaspoon ground cinnamon, and 1/2 teaspoon sea salt.

Stir until well hot and properly mixed.

3. Include Glaze:

Add the pineapple and nut mixture to the blender along with the honey-cinnamon glaze.

Incorporate the glaze into the smoothie by briefly blending.

4. Present and Garnish:

Transfer the blended drink to a bowl.

Add extra pineapple chunks, coconut flakes, or a dash of cinnamon as garnish.

5. Savor Your Morning Energy:

Start your day with a delicious and nutrient-rich smoothie bowl.

Day 1–7 (First Week): Smoothie Bowl for Evening Indulgence

1. Repetition of the Morning Routine

Make the morning smoothie bowl recipe for a satisfying and delicious dessert in the evening.

Day 8–14 (Week 2): Maintain the Schedule but Add Some Variation

1. Keep Things Consistent:

Make the slight modifications as necessary to the smoothie bowl recipes for the morning and evening.

Add some ice cubes for a cool variation.

Week 3, Days 15–21: Last Week of Nourishment

1. Adhere to the Schedule:

For breakfast and dinner, keep adding your nutrient-dense ingredients to the smoothie bowls.

2. Reflect on Your Travels:

Think for a moment on the ways in which this nutrient-dense practice has improved your health.

Extra Guidance

You can adjust the sweetness by adding more or less honey to suit your tastes.

Feel free to experiment with various toppings, such as sliced bananas, granola, or chia seeds, for some added variation.

Note: The purpose of this regimen is to add flavor and nutrition to your daily meals. It can be customized to fulfill dietary needs and individual tastes in order to support overall health.

5.3 Snacking on a Healthful Snack

1. Choose Your Time:

Whether it's an early morning boost, an afternoon pick-me-up, or a satisfying evening treat, choose a time that fits for your schedule.

2. Be Aware When You Prepare:

Collect the following ingredients: sea salt, crushed cinnamon, cashew nuts, peanuts, coconut flakes, honey, and coconut oil. Take your time assembling them all.

3. Establish a Calm Environment:

Choose a cozy spot where you can enjoy your smoothie bowl in silence and foster a contemplative eating experience.

4. incorporate with caution:

Blend pineapple, almonds, and honey-cinnamon glaze according to the recipe's directions to create a silky smooth blend. Permit your senses to be drawn in by the aromas.

5. Creative Garnishing

To improve the appearance, add more pineapple chunks, coconut flakes, or a touch of cinnamon to the garnish.

6. A Plateful of Joy:

Take your time and enjoy the contrast between the tropical sweetness and nutty richness with every spoonful.

7. Honoring the Nutrients:

Think about all the health benefits of each ingredient, including the vitamins in pineapple and the essential fats in almonds.

8. Consciously Consuming Food:

Savor the flavors, scents, and textures to arouse your senses. Allow each bite to be a deliberate delight.

Adapt to Your Choices

9. Adjust the Recipe:

You can experiment with different toppings, adjust the sweetness, or even try something new like adding ice cubes for a refreshing touch.

10. Spread the Happiness:

Serve this delicious smoothie to friends and family and consider creating a fun and healthful shared experience.

11. Consider your wellbeing:

After you've completed your meal, take a moment to appreciate the energy you've given your body and the satisfaction of a nutritious beverage.

12. Rehydrate and hydrate:

Drink something cold, like water or herbal tea, with your smoothie bowl to stay hydrated and enhance the whole experience.

Note: While enjoying a nutrient-rich snack, it's equally vital to cultivate a thoughtful and health-conscious eating routine. Embrace the nourishing pleasure that comes with each delicious bite.

In summary

After all of our research on the nutrient-dense Honey-Glazed Pineapple and Nut Smoothie Bowl, it is evident that this dish is more than simply a meal; rather, it is a sensory experience that combines taste, health, and mindful eating. Carefully crafted, this delicious and nutritious blend includes fresh pineapple, cashew nuts, peanuts, coconut flakes, honey, and coconut oil flavored with cinnamon.

We've grown to love not just the sweet delight of tropical fruits but also the complex flavors and essential minerals found in coconut and nuts as we've been savoring every bite. The careful preparation and eating of this smoothie bowl promote awareness of the connection between flavor, aroma, and well-being.

Our culinary adventure has inspired us to slow down and express our gratitude for the food that nature has so kindly given us. The thrill of personalization transforms this nutritious dish into something truly distinctive, whether it's adjusting the sweetness or trying different topping combinations.

As you include it into your daily routine, let this nutritious fruits-shake serve as a reminder that being healthy is a holistic process. Eating mindfully promotes a positive relationship with food in addition to its health benefits. A nutrient-dense smoothie bowl can become a ritual that honors self-care, health consciousness, and the fulfillment that comes from providing your body with what it needs.

So let each bowlful be a treasured memory, an enjoyable diversion from the day, and a delicious method to demonstrate your commitment to good health. I hope that learning about nutrition and taste would encourage healthy snacking habits that will eventually lead to a livelier and more satisfying lifestyle.

Encouraging people to make informed decisions is crucial since sexual health is an integral part of overall well-being. By embracing the truth, dispelling myths, and encouraging open dialogue, we contribute to a culture that recognizes sexual health as a necessary component of a happy and healthy life.

1. Comprehensive Sexual Education: Providing thorough sexual education is the first step in promoting informed opinions. This education should cover consent, respectful interactions, and emotional well-being in addition to the physical aspects of sexual health.

2. Overcoming Taboos and Stigmas: It's critical to address taboos and cultural stigmas around sexual health. Honest talks remove myths and create an environment where individuals feel comfortable asking for knowledge and assistance without fear of being condemned.

3. Promoting Diversity: It's critical to recognize and value a variety of sexual identities, orientations, and experiences.

An inclusive approach fosters a sense of welcome and belonging by making sure that resources and information are customized to meet each person's unique needs.

4. Evidence-Based Sexual Health Education: In sexual health education, it is imperative to emphasize material that is supported by research. People can make well-informed decisions when they possess full knowledge, which is helped by reliable sources, empirical research, and professional assistance from medical specialists.

5. Dispelling Myths and Irrational Beliefs: It is everyone's responsibility to dispel myths around sexual health. By dispelling myths, we contribute to a society that values truth above false beliefs, so reducing the likelihood of harmful behaviors and promoting positive attitudes toward sexual health.

6. Promoting Regular Health Check-ups: Regular health check-ups, which include sexual health screenings, are a good way to encourage proactive treatment. Frequent examinations promote early issue detection, ensure timely response, and maintain overall health.

7. Creating Safe Spaces for Conversation: It's important to create spaces that are safe for sincere dialogue. Conversation platforms allow people to engage with others, ask questions, and receive assistance in a variety of settings, including healthcare, education, and community forums.

8. Respect for Autonomy and Consent: Encouraging enthusiastic consent and upholding individual liberty are the cornerstones of sexual health. Positive reinforcement of boundaries, wants, and expectations fosters wholesome, consenting partnerships.

9. Information Empowerment: Knowledge is a powerful tool for empowerment. Providing people with appropriate sexual health information enhances their ability to make decisions that align with their values, interests, and overall well-being.

10. Celebrating Healthy Relationships: Promoting partnerships that prioritize communication, mutual respect, and trust contributes to the development of a culture that supports sexual health. Healthy connections are essential for both overall life satisfaction and emotional well-being.

It takes a team effort to promote informed perspectives on sexual health, including societal attitudes, education, and communication. We enable individuals to take charge of their sexual health journeys with agency, knowledge, and confidence by fostering an environment that values candid information, acknowledges and respects different viewpoints, and prioritises open communication.

www.ingramcontent.com/pod-product-compliance
Lightning Source LLC
Chambersburg PA
CBHW050838260726

48660CB00006B/2316